FIGHTING ADDICTION

A Powerful Book to Prevent You from Relapse

Michelle Gold

TABLE OF CONTENTS

CHAPTER 1

INTRODUCTION

Having a better understanding concerning the word "Addiction", several pictures or footage come back to our mind. We tend to see a girl World Health Organization sells her body in exchange for a "fix. We tend to see the falling down drunk "we tend to keep in mind a drunken disabled man on a wheel a chair owing to a drunk-driving accident. We tend to examine a known mortal World Health Organization died, and another whose sensational sex scandals area unit splashed across the tabloids. Most people grasp a lover or loved one, whose lives are a unit littered with addiction. We tend to all grasp that addiction may be a major problem. However, behind that wide command agreement area unit several disagreements and queries. However huge area unit addiction issues exactly?

However will addiction disagree from experimentation, wrongdoing, and dangerous habits? What causes addiction? However do you overcome it? However productive is addiction treatment? However ought to society reply to people with addiction? What ought to governments do concerning addiction? Is addiction principally a contemporary drawback? Is that the addiction problem obtaining worse?

Article won't resolve all the ardent debates encompassing these queries. With such a lot conflict and variations of opinion, it's usually troublesome to separate truth from opinion, and story from reality. Therefore, our goal is additional modest: to assist you, the reader; gain a stronger understanding of this advanced issue so you'll find your own opinions concerning addiction. During this method, if you or somebody you're keen on is combating Associate in nursing addiction drawback, you'll build Associate in nursing hip call concerning what to try and do concerning it.

CHAPTER 2

WHAT IS ADDICTION?

Addiction may be an advanced illness, typically chronic in nature that affects the functioning of the brain and body. It conjointly causes serious injury to families, relationships, schools, workplaces and neighborhoods. The foremost common symptoms of addiction area unit severe loss of management, continued use despite serious consequences, preoccupation with victimization, failing tries to quit, tolerance and withdrawal. Addiction are often effectively prevented, treated and managed by care professionals together with family or peer support.

More so, Addiction may be an advanced condition, an encephalopathy that's manifested by compulsive substance use despite harmful consequence. Individuals with addiction (severe substance use disorder) have associate intense concentrate on employing a bound substance(s), like alcohol or medication, to the purpose that it takes over their life. They keep victimization alcohol or a drug even after they realize it can cause issues. Nevertheless variety of effective treatments area unit on the market and folks will get over addiction and lead traditional, productive lives.

CHAPTER 3

WHAT PEOPLE ARE ADDICTED TOO

ADDICTION TO GAMBLING;

Constantly bucking your odds? Of all behavioral addictions, associate addiction to gambling is that the one that almost all closely resembles drug and white plague. The Yankee medical specialty Association (APA) classifies gambling disorder as associate habit forming disorder. Studies show that gambling addictions illuminate constant areas of the brain as drug addictions and treatment for gambling disorder is sometimes enclosed within the same style of medical care settings as drug and substance abuse.

ADDICTION TO SEX;

You often hear a couple of people going into rehab for sex addiction; however is a fanatical looking for sex a true addiction? Perhaps: though it is not formally classified as associate addiction, there are treatments for it, and also the APA did take into account, but reject, the concept of adding habit-forming sexual behavior to the fifth edition of its Diagnostic and applied math Manual of Mental Disorders underneath the heading "hypersexual behavior disorder." additionally, the symptoms of sex addiction together with loss of management and disrespect for risks and consequences are terribly just like those of ancient addictions. What is a sex addict to do? Like medicine, alcohol, and even gambling, hypersexual activity appears to reply best to 12-step programs, like Sex Addicts Anonymous.

ADDICTION TO INTERNET¿

We're living in a much wired world however is it attainable to be too obstructed in? Psychologists and psychiatrists do not typically take into account web addiction a real addiction. However it is often a haul for a few folks once it involves loss of management, in addition as negative consequences at work and reception. Analysis given at the 2014 annual meeting of the yank psychiatrically Association perceived to support the concept of web addiction by showing changes within the brain known by neuroimaging. The net could occupy up to eleven hours out of associate "Internet addict's" day. Studies recommend that compulsive web use affects half-dozen to fourteen percent of web users.

ADDICTION TO FOOD;

For the past decade, there is argument over whether or not food obsessions can actually be food addictions, or whether or not this "disorder" is a lot more of an excuse. In truth, binge upset could be a real downside that affects concerning three % of adults within the world. Symptoms embrace uptake to ease emotions, overdoing it on food whereas alone, and feeling guilty once the binge. The reason for uptake disorders isn't better known; however it's most likely connected a lot of to depression than addiction.

ADDICTION TO SHOPPING;

Shopping: It's yet one more behavior that, once it spins out of management, is taken into account to be associate impulse management disorder (rather than a real addiction). Does one purchase things to avoid feeling unhappy on the other hand feel guilty afterwards? Does one have a closet jam-packed with garments that also have the worth tags on them? You may be a shopper. Studies show that compulsive looking affects additional ladies than men, whom it may end up in massive issues, each financially and in person. However are you able to get help? Treatment for a looking addiction typically involves content and activity medical aid.

ADDICTION TO DRUG;

Drug addiction, conjointly known as substance use disorder, could be an ailment that affects somebody's brain and behavior and results in an inability to regulate the employment of a legal or embezzled drug or medication. Substances like alcohol, marijuana and alkaloid are also thought-about medication. Once you are addicted, you will continue exploitation the drug despite the damage it causes.

Drug addiction will begin with experimental use of a narcotic in social things, and, for a few individuals, the drug use becomes additional frequent. For others, significantly with opoids, dependence begins with exposure to prescribed medications, or receiving medications from an admirer or relative World Health Organization has been prescribed the medication.

The risk of addiction and the way quick you become addicted varies by drug. Some drugs, like opioid painkillers, have the next risk and cause addiction additional quickly than others.

As time passes, you would like larger doses of the drug to induce high. Shortly you will like the drug simply to feel sensible. As your drug use will increase, you will notice that it's progressively troublesome to travel while not the drug. Makes an attempt to prevent drug use could cause intense cravings and cause you to feel physically sick (withdrawal symptoms).

You may like facilitate from your doctor, family, friends, support teams or AN organized treatment program to beat your dependence and keep sober.

ADDICTION TO ALCOHOL;

If you have got a bit an excessive amount of alcohol once during whereas, it most likely won't do lasting injury if you're otherwise healthy. However it's a unique story if you often drink heavily.

For most men, that's outlined as over four drinks each day, or fourteen or fifteen during a week. For women, serious drinking is over three drinks during a day, or seven or eight per week.

Too much alcohol will damage you physically and mentally in various ways which include liver damage, anemia, brain and nervous system disorder, and cancer in most cases.

So, it is advisable to think closely before taking any decision that can damage the body and further damage one's life.

CHAPTER 4

MISUSE OF SUBSTANCES

Drug addiction and drug misuse square measure completely different.

Misuse refers to the wrong, excessive, or non-therapeutic use of body- and psychoactive substances.

However, not a soul that misuses a substance has Associate in nursing addiction. Addiction is that the long inability to moderate or stop intake.

For example, someone UN agency drinks alcohol heavily on an evening out might expertise each the euphoria and harmful effects of the substance.

However, this doesn't qualify as Associate in Nursing addiction till the person feels the necessity to consume this quantity of alcohol often, alone, or now and then of day once the alcohol can possible impair regular activities, like within the morning.

A person UN agency has not nonetheless developed Associate in Nursing addiction could also be shelve additional use by the harmful facet effects of drug abuse. For instance, disgorgement or awakening with a hangover when drinking an excessive amount of alcohol might deter some individuals from drinking that quantity anytime presently.

Someone with Associate in nursing addiction can still misuse the substance in spite of the harmful effects.

CHAPTER 5

SYMPTOMS TO NOTE THAT ONE HAS REACHED THE LEVEL OF ADDICTION

The primary indications of addiction are:

Uncontrollably seeking medication

Uncontrollably partaking in harmful levels of addictive behavior

Neglecting or losing interest in activities that don't involve the harmful substance or behavior

Relationship difficulties, which regularly involve lashing out at people that determine the dependency

Associate degree inability to prevent employing a drug, although it's going to be inflicting health issues or personal issues, like problems with employment or relationships

Concealing substances or behaviors and otherwise physical exercise secrecy, for instance, by refusing to elucidate injuries that occurred whereas below the influence

Profound changes in look, as well as an evident abandonment of hygiene

Accrued risk-taking, each to access the substance or activity and whereas mistreatment it or partaking in it

CHAPTER 6

TREATMENT TO ADDICTION

It is best for you to notice that healthful advances and progress in designation have helped the medical profession develop numerous ways that to manage and resolve addiction.

Methods include:

• Behavioral medical aid and content

- Medication and drug-based treatment

- Medical devices to treat withdrawal

- treating connected psychological factors, like depression

- Ongoing care to scale back the chance of relapse

Addiction treatment is extremely customized and infrequently needs the support of the individual's community or family.

Treatment will take an extended time and will be sophisticated. Addiction could be a chronic condition with a spread of psychological and physical effects. Every substance or behavior could need completely different management.

CHAPTER 7

DON'T JUST BELIEF, TAKE ACTION

Since religion and non secular beliefs will facilitate folks address addiction, actions impressed by spirituality or faith may be helpful to recovery. One such act is service to others. Service to others address their addictions, or serving to others in any manner, will facilitate improve a person's confidence and shallowness. Serving others may facilitate folks shift their focus off from their own struggles and urges, if solely quickly. This can be a primary element of the 12 step model, also, as cluster members are inspired to support one another and reach bent those that would like facilitate.

Another action that is additionally a part of you and that is to hunt forgiveness from others. Reaching bent those that were hurt by the addiction will facilitate mend broken relationship and increase the amount of positive relationships for social support. Sometimes, folks in recovery may get pleasure from forgiving people who have hurt them. This not solely mends some relationships, it may facilitate folks overcome negative thoughts and emotions concerning others.

THE END